Family Addictus

A New Understanding of Addiction, Recovery, and the Stories That Shape Us

Joe Van Wie

AllBetter Media

Copyright © 2025 by Joe Van Wie

All rights reserved. Published by AllBetter Media.

No portion of this book may be reproduced in any form without written permission from the publisher or author, except as permitted by U.S. copyright law.

ISBN (Print): 979-8-9998102-0-5
ISBN (Ebook): 979-8-9998102-1-2

Contents

Preface	1
Introduction	2
Part I: The Roots of Addiction	4
1. Addiction Is an Adaptation	5
2. The First 1,000 Days	8
3. Dopamine, Cortisol, and the Hijacked Brain	12
4. Attachment Styles and Emotional Tuning	17
5. Trauma is the Architect	21
Part II: Family Systems, Survival, and Society	25
6. Family Addictus: A Species-Level Phenomenon	26
7. Culture as Software, the Brain as Hardware	30

8. Disembodiment, Technology, and the Post-Labor World	34
9. Connection as the Antidote to Trauma	37
Part III: Recovery as Awakening	41
10. How Recovery Reclaims the Frontal Lobe	42
11. The Twelve CORES of Fellowship House	45
12. From Survival to Spiritual Awakening	50
Acknowledgments	55
About the Author	57
Appendix A: Glossary	59
Appendix B: Recommended Reading and Resources	63
Appendix C: Family Support Resources	67
Appendix D: The Twelve CORES (Expanded)	69
Appendix E: Fellowship House Experiences	73

Preface

Four billion years ago, life began on Earth. And although we don't know exactly how or where (scientists have theories about alkaline vents and ancient ice), every living thing on this planet shares the same origin. Your DNA connects you to oak trees and orcas, to bacteria and blue whales. There's only one tree of life, and we're all on it together.

This connection isn't just biological. It's the foundation of everything we'll explore in this book. Addiction thrives on the illusion that we're separate, that our pain is uniquely ours, that we're fundamentally alone. Recovery happens when we remember that we are part of something larger.

Family Addictus is about waking up to that connection. Not just to other people, but to the shared human experience of suffering, healing, and finding our way back to each other.

Introduction

In this book, we will cover topics that range from biology to psychology to spirituality. We'll discuss moral evolution, attachment styles, neuroplasticity, dopamine production, trauma theory, interpersonal relationships, language and myths. There are hundreds of books devoted to any of these topics—if you want a deeper dive, I've provided a list of works in the resources section, and there's endless information accessible online.

The point of this book is to take all these disparate concepts and weave them together into one narrative: the narrative of addiction. When placed in context, ideas that can seem overly complex and difficult to understand become simpler and digestible. Having a high-level understanding of addiction and all of its components is tremendously helpful to anyone seeking recovery or the family members of those who suffer from addiction.

At Fellowship House, we've learned that addiction is never just about the substance. It's about what happened before the first drink, the relationships that shaped us, the culture that made disconnection feel normal, and the brain that adapted to survive. This book maps that territory—not to explain addiction away, but to help you understand how healing becomes possible when we see the whole picture.

To learn more, visit fellowshiphouses.com and allbetter.fm.

Part 1: The Roots of Addiction

Addiction Is an Adaptation

Something was missing from the beginning, but you couldn't name what. Your parents weren't cruel, maybe just stressed, distracted, overwhelmed. But your nervous system knew. It was scanning for safety that never quite arrived. You only felt that missing piece later in life when a drink, a drug, or a behavior landed in your body and whispered, *There it is*. Something had arrived that felt like it should have always been there.

Most people call this addiction. It's actually an adaptation.

Addiction is the brain's answer to a deeper question. It arrives not as the first problem, but often as the first solution. The first way something finally works. For a person whose early emotional landscape was chaotic, under-attuned, or hypervigilant, substances or compulsive behaviors become predictable, controllable sources of comfort and relief. In a world that often felt unsafe or inconsistent, addiction becomes a map.

The Survival Brain

We're wired for survival, not logic. When your brain detects a threat, real or imagined, it doesn't care about your five-year plan. It wants relief, and it wants it now. The midbrain, which handles survival responses like fight, flight, and freeze, can hijack logical thinking when danger feels near. In addiction, this emergency mode becomes the default setting. The brain chooses relief over reason. Safety over strategy. Dopamine becomes the guide.

Picture a caveman running from a predator. In that moment, their brain isn't thinking about five-year plans or existential crises. It's looking for an escape hatch. Now imagine that same neurological response being triggered not by a tiger, but by being left on read, by a parent who never makes eye contact, by silence after trauma.

When the alarm bells go off too often, the brain adapts. It begins to build roads toward relief. And some roads are fast: nicotine, alcohol, porn, gambling, meth, rage, control, codependency. They become the express lanes to a different state of being.

Shiva's Dream

In Hindu mythology, the god Shiva falls asleep and dreams the world into existence. In this dream, he becomes us: forgetful, reactive, afraid. The story is a metaphor for waking up. For remembering. Recovery is much like this: a realization that we have been sleepwalking, that the ego, a protector built from years of emotional data, has been running the show.

Addiction is not a moral failure. It is a logical conclusion drawn by an emotional and evolutionary brain trying to survive a confusing, often painful environment. The substance is not the problem. The substance is the answer to a problem we have yet to name.

Recovery is the naming.

The First 1,000 Days

If addiction is an adaptation, then we must ask: what exactly are we adapting to?

The answer often begins in a time we don't consciously remember: the first 1,000 days of life. From in utero to age two, the human brain undergoes its most rapid development. This period doesn't just lay the foundation for motor skills or language. It sets the emotional tone of our nervous systems. Our capacity for self-regulation, trust, connection, and safety is shaped here, not through words, but through attunement.

What Is Attunement?

Attunement is like tuning a guitar, not to play alone, but to be in harmony with others. When a caregiver mirrors a baby's emotional cues through eye contact, facial expression, tone of voice, and physical comfort, they are sending a signal: you are safe here. This rhythm, repeated thousands of times a day, wires the brain for connection.

But when attunement is inconsistent, absent, or chaotic, the child's emotional system doesn't learn harmony. It learns vigilance. Even in loving homes, if the parent is preoccupied, depressed, anxious, overworked, or under-supported, that child may begin life emotionally out of tune. And like a musician playing to the wrong key, everything feels slightly off. The world is noisy. Internal chaos becomes the norm.

This isn't abuse in the traditional sense. It's often invisible. Subtle. Cultural. A working mother in her third trimester who's exhausted but unsupported. A father who's present but emotionally closed. A house that's clean but heavy with unspoken conflict. These are the early environments where misattunement begins, not through cruelty, but through stress, distraction, or inherited pain.

Cortisol vs. Dopamine

When the environment around a child is unpredictable or emotionally distant, the brain responds with cortisol, the stress hormone. Elevated cortisol levels during these early years can suppress dopamine production, which is crucial for pleasure, motivation, and learning. Over time, the child may grow into an adult who cannot feel good naturally, who struggles with sleep, self-soothing, or emotional regulation.

So when that person meets a substance—nicotine, cannabis, sugar, sex—it's not just a vice. It feels like a missing piece has finally arrived. It produces dopamine the brain never learned to make on its own. It fills a neurochemical absence that began long before the person ever made a conscious choice.

The Infant as Mirror

A newborn is not just a body. They are a mirror. Their earliest sense of identity comes not from within, but from what is reflected to them. If the mirror is cracked, if caregivers are emotionally unavailable or inconsistent, the child doesn't see a coherent self. They feel fragmented, anxious, or even invisible. And they begin building an identity to survive, not to thrive.

This is the seed of the adaptive self: the protector, the pleaser, the controller, the rebel, the perfectionist. Each one is a strategy to get the dopamine that never came freely.

Naming the Invisible

By the time addiction enters the picture, the original wound may be unrecognizable. The person might say, "I had a great childhood," because there was no overt trauma. But inside, they are dysregulated, lonely, driven by invisible hungers. These are the fingerprints of early misattunement.

Naming this matters. Not to blame parents or caregivers, but to break the spell. To understand that addiction is not a failure. It is an adaptation to an environment where emotional nourishment was scarce, and the brain had to get creative about survival.

Dopamine, Cortisol, and the Hijacked Brain

Think of your brain as a city. There are highways and alleyways, traffic lights and emergency sirens, and a central command center overseeing it all. But when stress becomes chronic or trauma goes unresolved, the sirens never stop. The traffic lights are always blinking red. And eventually, the backroads become shortcuts to the same dead end: escape.

This is the architecture of the addicted brain.

Addiction is not a flaw in moral reasoning. It is a feedback loop between survival systems and a hijacked reward system, orchestrated by three major players: dopamine, cortisol, and the midbrain.

Dopamine: The Anticipation Chemical

Contrary to popular belief, dopamine isn't the chemical of pleasure. It's the chemical of pursuit. It doesn't say "that felt good." It says, "go get it again."

In healthy brains, dopamine helps motivate us toward food, connection, achievement, and creativity. In misattuned or traumatized brains, where natural sources of safety and satisfaction were scarce or unpredictable, dopamine gets redirected. It gets hijacked by fast-acting substances and behaviors that flood the system with false rewards.

This is why the first cigarette or drink feels like magic. It doesn't just offer relief. It creates the illusion of arrival.

Over time, though, the dopamine system becomes desensitized. The same behaviors no longer produce the same effect. More is needed for less reward. This is not about poor choices. This is about chemistry doing what it was designed to do: adapt.

Cortisol: The Alarm Bell

Cortisol is the brain's primary stress hormone. It's not inherently bad. It wakes you up in the morning and helps you survive danger. But chronic exposure, especially in the first 1,000 days or during extended stress periods, keeps the alarm bell ringing long after the fire is out.

High cortisol shrinks the hippocampus (memory) and enlarges the amygdala (fear center), creating a brain that's always on edge. It also suppresses dopamine production. The end result? A person who feels chronically unsafe and chemically unable to experience joy.

The Midbrain: Where Survival Lives

When stress is high and dopamine is low, the midbrain takes over. It's the seat of instinct, drive, and habit. It's designed to act fast and doesn't bother with reflection. It doesn't weigh pros and cons. It asks only: Will this relieve the threat now?

This is why people in active addiction often describe their behavior as automatic. They aren't lying. They aren't making excuses. Their executive function (prefrontal cortex) is offline. The midbrain is driving.

And what relieves the threat the fastest? Substances that increase dopamine and suppress cortisol, even if only for minutes.

Addiction as a Neurochemical Loop

This triad of high cortisol, low dopamine, and midbrain dominance forms a loop:

    1. Stress or unresolved emotion triggers

cortisol.

2. Cortisol dampens dopamine.

3. Low dopamine increases cravings for external relief.

4. Substance use spikes dopamine, providing temporary relief.

5. The brain remembers this shortcut and repeats the cycle.

The longer this loop runs, the more it becomes the default setting. Like ruts in a road, these pathways deepen until they seem like the only available route.

But these patterns are not permanent, because the brain has neuroplasticity. Which means that with safety, connection, therapy, and time, it can be rewired.

At Fellowship House, we help clients:
- Engage the prefrontal cortex through CBT and narrative therapy.

- Calm the amygdala through mindfulness and emotional attunement.

- Reignite dopamine systems through authentic relationships and meaningful experiences.

Understanding this neurochemical loop helps explain why willpower alone rarely works. The midbrain doesn't respond to logic—it responds to safety, connection, and new experiences that can slowly retrain the reward system.

Attachment Styles and Emotional Tuning

You're born as an instrument. You don't know how to play yet, but you're already being tuned. The hands doing the tuning belong to your caregivers, and whether they are consistent, harsh, absent, or warm, their presence sets your tone. This is the essence of attachment: the emotional key in which we learn to play.

Attachment theory helps us understand why some people feel secure in relationships and others feel like they're always holding their breath. It explains why some of us reach for others in panic, while others pull away to survive. These patterns aren't flaws but adaptations to the emotional environment of our earliest years.

The Four Attachment Styles

Secure Attachment

When caregivers are attuned, predictable, and responsive, children develop a secure base. These individuals grow up trusting relationships, self-regulating emotions, and navigating stress with resilience. In adulthood, they can ask for help without shame. They don't fear closeness or independence. Recovery often comes more naturally to them because connection isn't terrifying.

Anxious Attachment

Formed when caregivers are inconsistent, sometimes loving, sometimes distant. The child learns that love is unreliable and begins to fear abandonment. In adulthood, this manifests as clinging, codependence, or emotional volatility. These individuals may turn to substances when their emotional needs feel unmet or overwhelming.

Avoidant Attachment

Developed when caregivers are emotionally distant, hypercritical, or unresponsive. The child learns that showing emotion is risky and that connection is not safe. As adults, they may suppress their feelings, dismiss intimacy, and use substances as a private refuge from emotional discomfort. Recovery for them can be isolating and slow because connection feels like exposure.

Disorganized Attachment

Often the result of trauma or abuse, this style is a chaotic mix of approach and avoidance. The caregiver is both a source of comfort and fear. The nervous system never finds a stable rhythm. These individuals often have complex trauma, emotional dysregulation, and a high risk of substance use. Recovery requires intense safety and structure to begin to rebuild trust in any relationship, including the one with oneself.

The Emotional GPS

Attachment isn't just a psychological concept. It's a biological guidance system. From infancy, it wires the brain to seek safety, connection, and meaning. When attunement is missing, this GPS can send out mixed signals:

- Trust no one.

- You are too much.

- You have to earn love.

- You're safest alone.

Substances can feel like a recalibration. A way to get back in tune. But like using a faulty compass, they often lead us deeper into confusion.

Recovery as Retuning

Attachment patterns are not destiny but blueprints that can be reshaped with support, therapy, and healthy relationships.

At Fellowship House, we:

- Identify attachment patterns with our clients.

- Use narrative therapy to rewrite internal stories.

- Practice mindfulness and relational safety in groups.

- Encourage earned secure attachment through consistency and care.

Attachment explains why some people feel emptier when they get sober because the substance was the only "secure base" they ever had. It explains why some clients resist help because help once hurt them. And it helps everyone involved understand how to offer support without perpetuating harmful patterns.

Trauma is the Architect

If addiction is a house, trauma is often the architect.

Not the loud, obvious kind of trauma we recognize in movies, but more often the subtle kind that never got a name. The absence of safety, the silence after fear, the love that felt conditional, the day you stopped crying because it didn't seem to matter.

What Is Trauma?

Dr. Gabor Maté, a physician and trauma expert, defines trauma not as the thing that happened, but as what happens inside you as a result—not the event but the imprint that interrupts emotional development and freezes parts of the nervous system in survival mode.

It doesn't need to be abuse, but could be a parent who was chronically stressed, emotionally absent, or grieving, a school environment that shamed expression, an unstable home, a sibling with special needs, or a parent with untreated mental illness. Trauma doesn't always shout. Sometimes it whispers.

Trauma Lives in the Body

When something is too overwhelming to process, it doesn't just "go away" but gets stored in the body. The amygdala (our emotional smoke alarm) remembers, while the hippocampus (our contextual memory system) gets confused, and the body tightens, adapts, and braces as if the event is still happening.

Over time, the body becomes the story the mind tried to forget. Chronic tension, hypervigilance, digestive issues, shallow breathing, and emotional reactivity are often signs that trauma is still running the show.

Trauma sets off a feedback loop:

- A trigger (smell, tone, memory) reminds the nervous system of a past threat.

- The amygdala fires.

- Cortisol surges.

- The prefrontal cortex goes offline.

- The body prepares to fight, flee, or freeze.

This loop, repeated often enough, becomes a baseline. The person may seem calm on the outside, but inside, they're bracing for impact. Substances become a shortcut, not to feel good, but to feel less.

Addiction as Self-Protection

In this light, addiction isn't self-destruction but self-protection that went too far. It's the best strategy the nervous system could find when no better options felt available. It worked until it didn't.

Addiction becomes the body's way of saying: "I can't hold this alone. I need help, even if it hurts me."

Trauma-Informed Recovery

At Fellowship House, we don't ask, "What's wrong with you?" We ask, "What happened to you?" And even more importantly: "What story did your body tell itself after that?"

We work to:
- Identify and name the trauma without retraumatization.
- Help clients reconnect with the body safely.
- Rebuild the capacity to feel safe while feeling.

- Develop tools for regulation that don't rely on substances.

Somatic practices, EMDR, narrative therapy, and group work create space for the frozen parts to thaw. Healing begins not with analysis, but with presence.

Part II: Family Systems, Survival, and Society

Family Addictus: A Species-Level Phenomenon

Addiction doesn't happen in a vacuum but grows in context, wrapping itself around the environment like a vine. The first environment we all come from is family.

When we say "Family Addictus," we're not just talking about parents or siblings but about a biological, cultural, and relational system that shapes how we attach, regulate emotion, seek connection, and deal with pain.

The same way evolution gave us opposable thumbs and language, it also wired us for patterned emotional inheritance. When a family doesn't know how to metabolize fear, shame, or grief, those feelings get passed down not just through behavior, but through biology.

The Inheritance of Pain

You don't just inherit your grandfather's eyes but also his silence, his coping strategies, and his cortisol response. If his way of dealing with stress was to drink, yell, disappear, or disconnect—and no one ever talked about it—then that becomes the emotional software of the family, a virus in the code.

Sometimes, what we call addiction is a family-wide trauma adaptation where one person carries the symptoms, but the pain belongs to the system.

The Identified Patient

In family therapy, there's a term called the "identified patient"—the person who manifests the symptoms, the addict, the black sheep, the troubled teen. But they are often expressing a larger dysfunction that no one else can name.

It's like a fire alarm going off in a house that everyone insists isn't burning.

Healing begins when the family stops asking "Why can't you just stop?" and starts asking "What is this trying to tell us about our system?"

The Family as an Emotional Ecosystem

Just like an ecosystem, families can be resilient or fragile. Some are rich with emotional nutrients like safety, presence, and forgiveness, while others are nutrient-poor, filled with performance, avoidance, secrets, and suppression.

Addiction can be seen as a symptom of emotional drought where the substance becomes the fastest-growing weed in a garden where emotional nourishment is scarce.

Rewriting the Family Code

At Fellowship House, we believe families aren't just part of the problem but also part of the solution. We treat addiction as a family phenomenon because it spreads in relationships, is maintained through patterns, and can only fully heal when the system transforms.

That's why we invite families into the treatment process early, offer psychoeducation on attachment and generational trauma, help families write cost letters that share truth without shame, and guide systems toward shared reality and emotional honesty.

The Species-Level View

Step back far enough, and addiction becomes less about substances and more about human pain, misunderstood and inherited. It becomes a mirror of culture, class, and how we relate to vulnerability.

In this way, addiction isn't just a family disease but a species condition—a byproduct of consciousness meeting fear, a survival mechanism in a world that forgot how to sit with discomfort.

Recovery, at its best, is a relational awakening where a family learns a new language and a species remembers that it was built for connection.

Culture as Software, the Brain as Hardware

Think of your brain as a computer. From birth, it's a powerful machine with infinite potential, but it still needs one thing to operate: software.

That software is culture.

We don't just inherit eye color or temperament but also belief systems, unspoken rules, narratives about success and failure, strengths and weaknesses. These are downloaded into us through language, stories, rituals, school, media, and religion. Culture doesn't just influence what we think—it influences how we think.

And sometimes, the software is corrupted.

The Broken Code

In cultures where value is tied to productivity, status, or stoicism, emotional honesty becomes a bug rather than a feature. If you're praised for achievement but punished for vulnerability, you learn to suppress discomfort rather than process it. If your culture worships individualism, you're taught to go it alone, and if your culture stigmatizes mental health, you're taught that asking for help is failure.

When the code is corrupted, addiction becomes an almost rational response. If the only emotions that are allowed are success or silence, substances become the secret operating system that lets you feel something real.

The Download Begins Early

From birth, our brains are shaped by our environment. Donald Hebb, a Canadian psychologist widely regarded as the father of neuropsychology, famously said, "Neurons that fire together, wire together." This means repeated emotional experiences shape the architecture of the brain. What fires? What gets rewarded? What gets ignored?

This is why a child who grows up in a household that avoids emotion may grow into an adult who avoids emotion—not because they want to, but because their brain never downloaded the pathways for safely expressing fear, sadness, or need.

Now layer onto that a society that reinforces disconnection, where digital performance replaces intimacy, curated images replace community, and hustle replaces rest. The result? A nervous system with nowhere to land, and a midbrain constantly scanning for escape routes.

Culture as an Operating System

Philosopher Nick Bostrom suggested we might be living in a simulation, while cognitive scientist Donald Hoffman argued that perception itself is an interface, not a mirror of reality. These ideas may sound philosophical, but they support something very simple: we don't see the world as it is; we see it as we've been trained to see it.

Culture is that training, writing the script, while addiction exploits the bugs.

When feelings are inconvenient, substances become therapists. When speed is rewarded, stimulants become gods. When numbness is power, opioids become sacred. Addiction becomes both a personal struggle and a cultural symptom.

Rewriting the Code

Recovery requires both abstinence and a system reboot. At Fellowship House, we help clients examine their personal "operating systems," challenge inherited beliefs about worth, masculinity, success, failure, and connection, and develop new internal scripts rooted in compassion and curiosity.

Recovery asks: What code are you running? Who wrote it? Is it serving you? Healing the brain means rewriting the software that's been running the show.

Disembodiment, Technology, and the Post-Labor World

We used to live in our bodies. We worked with our hands, walked miles a day, felt the seasons on our skin. We gathered in circles, ate together, grieved together, danced, touched, and looked one another in the eyes.

Today, many of us live in our screens. We are more connected than ever yet less embodied, and this disconnection from the physical world, from our nervous systems, and from the felt reality of other people creates a perfect storm for addiction.

The Digital Nervous System

Technology has reprogrammed our instincts, replacing notifications for ritual, algorithms for intuition, and swipes for conversations. We now have dopamine on demand through infinite scroll, but what we gain in stimulation, we lose in regulation. The nervous system, built to process life through rhythm, breath, and presence, becomes overwhelmed by endless novelty. The frontal lobe (the seat of planning and reflection) gets constantly hijacked by reaction, while the body becomes a background prop we ignore until it breaks.

Addiction, in this context, becomes the brain's desperate attempt to anchor, to feel something real, to reclaim a center.

The Collapse of Purpose

At the same time, we are entering a new economic reality: the post-labor world. AI, automation, and algorithmic efficiency are replacing human roles faster than society can adapt. For many, especially the young, work no longer feels meaningful, and identity, once tied to vocation, now floats unmoored.

This collapse of traditional purpose fuels a quiet crisis: What am I for? What do I contribute? What makes life worth living? In that void, addiction flourishes because substances offer immediate purpose: numb the pain, quiet the question, repeat the loop.

When the Body Becomes Optional

In a disembodied world, the body is seen as optional since everything important happens online. Yet the body is where healing happens—recovery isn't digital but visceral.

As we navigate a future shaped by AI and post-labor economics, recovery must evolve too. We must create communities rooted in shared, physical space, offer purpose beyond productivity, and teach young people how to regulate before they medicate.

At Fellowship House, we bring people back to their bodies through breathwork, mindfulness, yoga, and somatic therapies, through group meals, eye contact, physical activity, and grounded conversation, and discomfort, which we learn to feel instead of escape.

Recovery means returning to reality: to the breath, to the body, to boredom, to beauty.

Connection as the Antidote to Trauma

If trauma is the wound, connection is the suture. Addiction isn't just a craving for a chemical but a longing for something we lost—or never had. Something felt, not seen. A sense of being with. Of safety in the presence of another nervous system that says: You're okay here.

The Social Brain

Humans are wired to connect. From birth, we seek attunement, eye contact, and co-regulation. Our brains are social organs, designed to light up in the presence of others. But when our early attempts at connection are met with rejection, absence, or chaos, we don't stop needing connection—we stop trusting it.

We adapt by self-soothing, disconnecting, and reaching for anything that mimics intimacy without risk. Substances, screens, gambling, sex, and achievement become synthetic stand-ins for what we truly want: to be known and still loved.

Isolation Is the Real Disease

British journalist Johann Hari, known for his work on addiction, famously said, "The opposite of addiction is not sobriety. It is connection." Isolation doesn't just worsen addiction—it fuels it.

Every relapse begins in subtle disconnection from community, from routine, from the body, from one's values. When people feel alone, their nervous systems become dysregulated, the midbrain takes over, and the body seeks relief.

Connection as Medicine

Real connection regulates the nervous system, restores rhythm, and tells the amygdala, "You're not alone. The danger has passed."

At Fellowship House, we cultivate connection through group therapy where vulnerability is welcomed, family programming where truths can be shared safely, peer relationships that foster trust and accountability, and staff who lead with empathy and shared experience.

Healing happens in a relationship, not in isolation. It happens when a client is seen in their grief and not turned away, when they share their shame and are still embraced, when they feel the presence of another person who says, "I've been there, and I'm not leaving."

What Connection Looks Like

Connection isn't just deep talks and tearful hugs, but can be laughing together in the kitchen, sitting quietly beside someone on a hard day, making eye contact and saying "Good morning," remembering someone's name, or noticing when someone withdraws and gently checking in.

Connection is attention, repeated over time.

Rewiring Through Relationship

The brain can change. Every time a client experiences a safe connection, a new pathway is laid and a new possibility is introduced.

Neuroscientist Bruce Hood has explored how the self and personality are not fixed traits but are shaped through experiences and interactions. In recovery, as clients begin to form secure relationships and participate in a culture of empathy, their personalities begin to change—not superficial shifts but deep reorganizations of the self, grounded in new neural wiring and social identity.

This aligns directly with what Alcoholics Anonymous describes as a "spiritual awakening": a fundamental change in personality that results from consistent participation in a shared recovery culture. Through sustained connection and mutual support, individuals begin to embody a new sense of self.

Over time, this becomes their new baseline where shame is replaced by acceptance, fear by trust, and loneliness by belonging. Connection is the treatment plan.

Part III: Recovery as Awakening

How Recovery Reclaims the Frontal Lobe

One of the most profound skills a person in recovery can learn isn't how to "fight" cravings but how to pause.

In the chaos of addiction, the midbrain—the part responsible for survival and impulse—takes control while logic, long-term thinking, and emotional balance get sidelined. The part of the brain built for presence and perspective, the prefrontal cortex, is overridden by instinct.

Recovery is the process of giving the frontal lobe the microphone again.

The Power of the Pause

This skill isn't just a recovery idea but a military one too. Navy SEALs are trained not to react, but to breathe, regulate, and assess. Under fire, they freeze—not in fear, but in awareness. They override the midbrain by activating the frontal lobe, where strategy lives.

The goal isn't to be fearless but to be conscious.

Autopilot vs. Awareness

Most people in active addiction describe doing things they swore they wouldn't do—not because they wanted to, but because it felt automatic. The neural loops were so deeply carved, the pause didn't exist. Craving. Use. Shame. Repeat.

This isn't about morality but about neurology.

Every time a person in recovery pauses—just long enough to ask, "Is this aligned with my values?" or "What will this feel like tomorrow?"—they are interrupting the old loop and forming a new one.

The Frontal Lobe Comes Online

When the prefrontal cortex is activated, we think long-term, regulate emotion, reflect, align with values, and slow down enough to choose. This is the seat of maturity, of recovery, of agency.

At Fellowship House, we train this through Cognitive Behavioral Therapy (CBT) to recognize distorted thinking and reframe it, mindfulness practices like breathing, noticing, and staying present, and narrative therapy to help clients observe their story instead of being stuck inside it.

Repetition Builds the Muscle

Pausing isn't natural at first, and for many, it feels like doing nothing. But it is doing the hardest thing: choosing not to react.

Like Navy SEALs rehearse under pressure, clients rehearse in groups. We talk about high-risk scenarios, write out the story before it happens, walk through the discomfort, and normalize the pause.

Over time, that pause becomes a gap, then the gap becomes a breath, then the breath becomes a choice. This is where freedom lives.

The Twelve CORES of Fellowship House

Recovery isn't just about abstinence but about building a life worth staying sober for.

At Fellowship House, we don't treat addiction like a temporary fire to be put out but as an invitation to rewire a whole life—a call to rebuild identity, purpose, and belonging from the ground up.

That's why we developed the Twelve CORES: a set of values, practices, and areas of growth that give structure to recovery and meaning to life beyond treatment. They are living principles that adapt to each person's story rather than rigid rules.

Think of recovery as a wheel where these CORES are its spokes. When they are strong, life rolls forward with balance and direction. When one is missing or weak, the wheel wobbles.

Or consider the brain as a hard drive that stores memory, emotion, instincts, and thought. Just like any computer, it needs software to run, and that software is culture. It tells the brain what to value, how to connect, what to fear, and how to interpret reality.

Unfortunately, most of us were handed corrupted software—systems built on shame, fear, disconnection, or performance. The CORES at Fellowship House act like a reformatting tool that reinstalls a new system based on connection, curiosity, and agency.

Like the swirling nickel-iron core of the Earth that generates a magnetic field to protect the planet from radiation, the CORES of recovery generate a kind of internal magnetism. When they are alive and active, they protect us from chaos, attract stability, and help life flourish.

Things can get complex in recovery, and life will always throw curveballs. But if your core is solid—anchored in something real—you have a superpower: a gravitational center, a moral compass, a blueprint for resilience.

The Twelve CORES of Fellowship House

Education: The Light of Understanding

Recovery begins with knowledge. Understanding the brain, trauma, addiction, and healing empowers people to participate fully in their transformation. Ignorance keeps us stuck; education sets us free.

Career (Vocation): Purpose and Contribution

Work gives structure and meaning. Whether it's a job, volunteering, or a creative pursuit, engaging with the world restores dignity and direction. Vocation isn't just a paycheck but an offering.

The Arts: Expression Beyond Words

Addiction suppresses the voice; the arts give it back. Painting, music, poetry, and storytelling allow clients to say what they couldn't put into words. Creativity is emotional fluency.

Family: Repairing the Bridge

The family is the patient. Whether it means reconnection, redefinition, or reconciliation, addressing the family system is essential for healing. Repair replaces blame while boundaries replace chaos.

Friendship: Building a New Tribe

Recovery requires belonging. We help clients cultivate relationships based on honesty, growth, and mutual support rather than old trauma bonds. We replace secrecy with sincerity.

Health: Mind, Body, and Spirit

We address nutrition, sleep, movement, and medical needs alongside emotional and spiritual health. Sobriety isn't wellness if the body is ignored. We teach the body to feel safe again.

Adventure: Rediscovering Play and Joy

We create experiences that reawaken wonder and pleasure: hiking, sports, travel, exploration. Clients learn that fun and freedom exist beyond substances. Joy becomes the medicine.

Altruism: The Gift of Giving Back

Service work changes the self. Helping others provides purpose and interrupts the isolation of addiction. Giving multiple meanings rather than depleting it.

Agency: The Return of Choice

We teach clients how to pause, reflect, and choose rather than react. Agency is the antidote to helplessness and the muscle that keeps growing. Freedom lives in the pause.

Ethos: Living with Integrity

Recovery isn't just about what you don't do but about who you are. We help clients define and live by their values. When behavior aligns with belief, shame dissolves.

Expertise: Trusting the Process

Recovery is complex. Our staff, many in recovery themselves, model lived experience with clinical skill. We lead with humility and credibility while experience becomes a bridge.

Individuality: Honoring the Unique Self

No two recoveries are alike. We celebrate the personal, spiritual, and cultural differences that make each story powerful. Authenticity is the goal rather than conformity.

A Living Culture of Recovery

These CORES aren't checklists but invitations. Recovery becomes a communal culture that reshapes identity, rewires connection, and restores meaning rather than just an individual journey.

From Survival to Spiritual Awakening

There is a moment in recovery that can't be forced, predicted, or perfectly described. It doesn't arrive with fireworks but often comes in silence, in stillness, a breath, a glance, a morning that doesn't start in panic, a moment of peace that feels unearned but real.

This is the beginning of spiritual awakening.

It has little to do with religion and everything to do with remembering who you are beneath the defenses, the masks, the cravings, and the chaos. It's about returning to what was always there rather than becoming someone new.

What Awakening Feels Like

It feels like agency, like breath, like forgiveness. It feels like the pause between stimulus and reaction, like walking away from a trigger instead of walking into it, like telling the truth when lying would be easier.

It feels like belonging to your own body again. Awakening doesn't mean you don't struggle, but that you struggle differently—with curiosity instead of contempt, with grace instead of shame.

Recovery Reorganizes the Self

To reduce addiction to simply a "brain disease" misses the mark for many. You are more than a brain—you are the software, too. You are the operating system and the conscious observer.

Your experience unfolds in the realm of consciousness, the unseen ether in which all brain activity takes place. We do not control all outcomes, and we cannot guarantee certainty. But we can tell you with confidence: this is the most stable and complete approach to recovery we have.

It acknowledges not just your neurobiology, but your story. It honors not just your symptoms, but your center of experience.

In the Twelve Steps of Alcoholics Anonymous, it is said that recovery is marked by a "spiritual awakening as the result of these steps." This concept of spiritual awakening was borrowed from the work of William James, often called the grandfather of modern psychology. In his seminal book *The Varieties of Religious Experience*

(1902), James explored the transformative nature of spiritual experiences, especially those that lead to a deep reorganization of character, perception, and purpose. His influence on the founders of AA—especially Bill Wilson—was profound. James posited that spiritual conversion could function as a legitimate psychological rebirth, marking a transition from despair to hope, from division to wholeness.

Neuroscientist Bruce Hood and others have pointed out that the "self" isn't a fixed entity but is emergent, relational, and a story in motion, shaped by memory, emotion, and culture.

Recovery, then, becomes about personality change—not in the sense of becoming someone else, but of reclaiming the self from outdated programming.

As the midbrain calms and the frontal lobe returns online, new choices become possible. As old beliefs are challenged, new narratives take shape. As the CORES become active, magnetism begins. The center holds.

The Side Effects of Awakening

A spiritual awakening doesn't just remove the need for substances but restores the natural side effects of a regulated, present, and empowered self:

Novelty returns, and life becomes interesting again. Curiosity replaces arrogance while the need to be right fades. Authenticity rises as help is received without effort, and vulnerability becomes natural. Connection deepens while people are seen as opportunities for cooperation rather than threats.

Awakening isn't about certainty but about humility and engaged participation in the human experience.

The Prefrontal Cortex: Home of Spiritual Life

The prefrontal cortex, often sidelined during addiction, is the brain's headquarters for long-term vision, moral decision-making, emotional regulation, and empathy. It is, in many ways, the neurological seat of the spiritual life.

And what is a spiritual life? A life of greater cooperation marked by service, sincerity, and harmony. A life where power is shared rather than hoarded. A life that ripples outward, quietly inviting others to rise.

The more we activate the prefrontal cortex, the more we embody these values as second nature rather than ideals.

Awakening Is Remembering

Many spiritual traditions echo this truth:

Shiva dreams the world and forgets he is dreaming. The Buddha awakens under a tree and sees clearly for the first time. Jesus withdraws to the desert, not to become someone else, but to remember the divine within.

Recovery joins this lineage as a waking up from the trance of survival, the sacred act of returning.

At Fellowship House, we don't give clients a destination but tools, space, safety, culture, and most importantly: connection. Dr. Viktor Frankl once wrote, "Between stimulus and response there is a space..." That space is where recovery begins. We believe awakening isn't a moment but a practice—a life lived from the inside out.

And so we end where we began. You are not broken. You adapted. You survived. And now, you are waking up.

Acknowledgments

This book is a collective memory, a constellation of insights, voices, and lessons that could never have been gathered alone.

To the staff at Fellowship House: your integrity, grit, compassion, and relentless commitment to building something beautiful amid pain gave this project its heartbeat. You didn't just show up for the work. You showed up for the people. You modeled recovery not as a concept, but as a culture.

To our alumni: thank you for trusting us with your stories. Thank you for returning, for checking in, for teaching us what recovery looks like after the discharge papers. Your voices are the roots of this book.

To Larry Moran Esq.: thank you for dreaming this place into being and for believing that clinical excellence and human warmth could coexist under one roof.

To Bruce Bicknell, aka "Santa Claus": your memory lives in every corner of this work. You taught me the holiness of presence, the power of laughter, and the courage it takes to keep showing up.

To the thinkers and healers who shaped this text—Dr. Gabor Maté, Dr. Bessel van der Kolk, William James, Bruce Hood, and the many clinicians who give voice to the science of what we've long felt in our bones: that healing is possible, and connection is the path.

To my family: thank you for letting me turn our pain into something that might help others. I carry your stories with reverence.

And finally, to the reader: if you found something in these pages that made you pause, reflect, or soften—thank you. This book belongs to you, too.

About the Author

Joe Van Wie (MSW, CADC) is a father, husband, filmmaker, speaker, and recovery advocate. He is the co-founder and CEO of Fellowship House in Scranton, Pennsylvania, a comprehensive PHP/IOP treatment program that serves individuals navigating the complex landscape of Substance Use Disorder.

A person in long-term recovery, Joe brings both lived experience and clinical insight to his work in the field. He believes recovery is about participation rather than perfection, and that healing begins when we stop asking, "What's wrong with you?" and start asking, "What happened to you, and who's walking with you now?"

Before entering recovery, Joe spent over a decade in the world of political strategy, advertising, and film. His award-winning feature, *Forged,* and his nationally recognized podcast AllBetter.fm reflect his lifelong passion for storytelling and creating space for truth.

Joe holds a Bachelor of Arts in Psychology from SUNY and has completed executive education in Artificial Intelligence and Leadership at MIT. He is currently completing his Master of Science in Social Work at Columbia University, where he continues to explore trauma, recovery, and systems change through a narrative and clinical lens.

Appendix A: Glossary

This glossary clarifies key terms used throughout *Family Addictus*. These definitions are simplified for accessibility and adapted for a recovery-informed audience.

Addiction. A chronic, patterned use of a substance or behavior despite negative consequences, often rooted in trauma, disconnection, and neurobiological adaptation.

Amygdala. A small, almond-shaped part of the brain that acts like an emotional smoke alarm. It detects threats and activates fight-or-flight responses.

Attunement. The process of being emotionally in sync with another person. In early childhood, attuned caregivers respond predictably and warmly to an infant's cues, laying the foundation for emotional regulation.

Attachment Style. Patterns of relating to others based on early experiences with caregivers. The four primary styles are secure, anxious, avoidant, and disorganized.

CBT (Cognitive Behavioral Therapy). A structured, evidence-based therapy that helps individuals identify and reframe negative thought patterns and behaviors.

Consciousness. The field of awareness in which thoughts, emotions, and experiences occur. The "ether" that holds our subjective sense of self.

Cortisol. The body's primary stress hormone. Useful in short bursts, but harmful when chronically elevated, as it suppresses dopamine and over-activates the fear response.

CORES (Fellowship House). Twelve domains of human growth have been identified as essential to long-term recovery: Education, Career, Arts, Family, Friendship, Health, Adventure, Altruism, Agency, Ethos, Expertise, and Individuality.

Dopamine. A neurotransmitter associated with motivation, pursuit, and reward. Often mischaracterized as the "pleasure chemical."

Disembodiment. The psychological detachment from the body. Common in trauma survivors and those living primarily in digital environments.

Frontal Lobe / Prefrontal Cortex. The brain region responsible for executive functioning, including long-term planning, emotional regulation, empathy, and impulse control. Seen here as the "seat of spiritual life."

Midbrain. The brain's survival center. Manages instinctual reactions and can override rational thought under stress.

Neuroplasticity. The brain's ability to change and rewire itself in response to experience, practice, and healing relationships.

Spiritual Awakening. A profound shift in perception and self-identity is often marked by increased awareness, connection, humility, and emotional coherence. Coined by AA and influenced by William James.

Trauma. Not just the event, but what happens inside you as a result of overwhelming experiences.

Trauma disrupts emotional development and alters brain chemistry.

William James. A philosopher and psychologist whose work, *The Varieties of Religious Experience*, deeply influenced modern understandings of spiritual transformation, especially in recovery culture.

Appendix B: Recommended Reading and Resources

This appendix includes key books, articles, podcasts, and films that inform the philosophy, clinical approach, and cultural reflections found in *Family Addictus*. These resources may deepen understanding for clients, families, clinicians, and curious minds.

Books

In the Realm of Hungry Ghosts by Dr. Gabor Maté. A foundational book exploring the link between trauma and addiction, emphasizing compassion over judgment.

The Body Keeps the Score by Dr. Bessel van der Kolk. Explores how trauma reshapes the body and brain and how healing requires reconnecting with the body.

The Varieties of Religious Experience by William James. Classic psychological work that helped shape the concept of spiritual awakening in recovery culture.

Chasing the Scream by Johann Hari. A compelling investigation into the roots of addiction and the importance of connection as a path to healing.

Lost Connections by Johann Hari. Focuses on depression and anxiety, emphasizing how disconnection fuels emotional suffering.

The Biology of Desire by Dr. Marc Lewis. A neuroscientist and former addict challenges the disease model, proposing that addiction is a learned response that can be unlearned.

The Addicted Brain by Dr. Michael Kuhar. A concise overview of how drugs affect the brain and how recovery is possible through brain-based change.

Unbroken Brain by Maia Szalavitz. Argues for a more compassionate and nuanced understanding of addiction as a learning disorder.

The Self Illusion by Bruce Hood. Explores how our sense of self is constructed by the brain and shaped by environment, supporting the idea that identity is malleable.

Podcasts

AllBetter.fm (hosted by Joe Van Wie). Features in-depth interviews with alumni, clinicians, advocates, and thought leaders in the field of recovery and mental health. Notable episodes include stories from Mike G., Amir, Joey, and Matt Ryan.

The Trauma Therapist Podcast (hosted by Guy Macpherson, PhD). A resource for those interested in the practice and process of trauma-informed care.

The Huberman Lab (hosted by Dr. Andrew Huberman). A science-based podcast exploring how neuroscience informs habits, recovery, and human potential.

Documentaries and Films

The Anonymous People (2013). Explores the stigma of addiction and the power of recovery advocacy.

Cracked Up (2019). Tells the story of comedian Darrell Hammond and the devastating impact of childhood trauma.

Pleasure Unwoven by Dr. Kevin McCauley. An award-winning film explaining the neuroscience of addiction using visual metaphors and clinical clarity.

Dosed (2019). Follows a woman with opioid addiction as she turns to psychedelic-assisted therapy.

Appendix C: Family Support Resources

Families are often the invisible carriers of addiction's weight. Healing together requires support, education, and permission to feel everything.

Trusted Organizations

Al-Anon Family Groups (al-anon.org). Support groups for anyone affected by someone else's drinking.

Nar-Anon Family Groups (nar-anon.org). For families and friends of those struggling with drug addiction.

Partnership to End Addiction (drugfree.org). Offers tools, helplines, and family-based guidance.

CRAFT (Community Reinforcement and Family Training). A non-confrontational, evidence-based approach to helping loved ones engage in treatment.

Books for Families

Beyond Addiction by Jeffrey Foote, Carrie Wilkens, and Nicole Kosanke.

It Takes a Family by Debra Jay.

Codependent No More by Melody Beattie.

Appendix D: The Twelve CORES (Expanded)

The Twelve CORES are a philosophy, a rhythm, a way of life rather than merely program elements. What follows is an expanded view into each CORE, how it shows up in recovery, and why it matters to the nervous system, to culture, and to the story we tell about ourselves.

1. **Education: The Light of Understanding.** Knowledge is empowerment. When clients understand how the brain works, how trauma impacts behavior, and how healing is possible, they begin to reclaim authorship over their story. Education interrupts shame and replaces it with insight.

2. **Career (Vocation): Purpose and Contribution.** Work gives rhythm, but vocation gives meaning. We don't just

help people get jobs—we help them discover what they are here to give. Contribution creates dignity while purpose replaces survival-mode functioning with future orientation.

3. **The Arts: Expression Beyond Words.** Words often fail where trauma lives. Music, painting, movement, and writing let the body speak its language. The arts are a mirror, a release, and a celebration. Creativity is coherence.

4. **Family: Repairing the Bridge.** No healing is complete without addressing the system that shaped us. We work with families to create new patterns rather than assign blame. Through honest conversation, boundaries, and cost letters, the bridge is rebuilt one plank at a time.

5. **Friendship: Building a New Tribe.** Addiction isolates, while recovery re-tribes. We emphasize shared experience, accountability, and fun. True friendship is one of the best relapse prevention tools available because it tells the brain: you're not alone anymore.

6. **Health: Mind, Body, and Spirit.** Nutrition stabilizes mood. Movement releases stored

trauma. Sleep heals the brain. Spiritual health fosters perspective. We treat health as a full-spectrum necessity rather than an afterthought.

7. **Adventure: Rediscovering Play and Joy.** Joy is the nervous system's natural reward. Hikes, excursions, and play remind the body that life without substances can be exhilarating. Adventure reactivates wonder and novelty—both essential to neuroplasticity.

8. **Altruism: The Gift of Giving Back.** Service repairs the ego. Helping others creates connection, meaning, and humility. Clients are invited to contribute to the community rather than just heal within it. Giving back is a graduation.

9. **Agency: The Return of Choice.** Agency is the antidote to victimhood. We teach pause, reflection, and decision. Every time a client chooses to respond instead of react, the frontal lobe strengthens. Agency creates dignity.

10. **Ethos: Living with Integrity.** Integrity is alignment—when our actions match our values. We help clients discover their moral compass and use it to navigate relationships,

work, and healing. Integrity breeds trust, within and without.

11. **Expertise: Trusting the Process.** Our staff are mentors, many with lived experience, rather than just professionals. Clients don't just learn from credentials but from people who have walked the same road. Expertise becomes relational rather than just informational.

12. **Individuality: Honoring the Unique Self.** Every recovery is different. We celebrate difference and challenge conformity. Identity is reclaimed rather than assigned. The client becomes the author of their story rather than just the character in someone else's narrative.

Appendix E: Fellowship House Experiences

These are real stories from clients, families, and clinicians whose lives intersected with Fellowship House. Names have been changed to protect anonymity where requested.

James P. "Before Fellowship House, I didn't know how to sit still. I thought addiction was just about stopping drugs. What I found here was a way to finally be in a room without needing to run from myself. The CORES gave me something I didn't even know I needed—a structure for becoming a man I actually like."

Mariah S. (Mother of Former Client). "Our son had been to four rehabs before this one. Fellowship House was the first place that treated our family like part of the healing rather than just spectators. The letters, the family sessions, the honesty—they saved our relationship."

Jerome W. "I came in angry. I thought recovery was a joke. What changed me wasn't some dramatic moment; it was the kitchen. The laughing. The way the staff remembered my name. I started trusting one person at a time. That's what made the cravings lose their power."

Elena T. (Clinician). "I've worked in mental health for 17 years. This program is the only one I've seen that integrates trauma, neuroscience, family work, and genuine cultural change under one roof. It's lived philosophy rather than just curriculum."

Marcus V. "I had no idea what it meant to have agency until I started learning about the frontal lobe and trauma. I used to think my past was just who I was. Here, I learned how to pause. That pause changed everything."

Tina L. "They didn't just teach me how to stay sober. They helped me learn how to live. I know who I am now. That's the real miracle."

Isaiah M. "The Fellowship House approach felt like someone finally handed me the manual for how my nervous system works. I got to stop blaming myself and start understanding myself. That saved my life."

To share your own story, please visit fellowshiphouses.com/testimonials.

For deeper dives into the recovery journeys of alumni like Mike G., Amir, Joey, and Matt Ryan, visit AllBetter.fm, Joe Van Wie's nationally recognized podcast in the field of addiction and mental health recovery.

For 24-hour addiction support call 1-888-HELP-121.

www.ingramcontent.com/pod-product-compliance
Lightning Source LLC
Chambersburg PA
CBHW020600030426
42337CB00013B/1153